lost weight 200 answer

by

RICHARD THE GREEN

contents

Chapter one

1:How can I lose 10 pounds in 7 days?

Here are the 6 steps you should follow in order to lose 10 pounds in a week.

1:Quickly Eat Fewer Carbs and More Lean Proteins.

2:Eat Whole Foods and Avoid Most Processed Junk Foods.

3:Reduce Your Calorie Intake .

4:Lift Weights and Try High-Intensity Interval Training.

5:Be Active Outside of the Gym.

6:Intermittent Fasting Is Another Simple Way to Reduce Weight.

2:What are the best diets for 2018?

Here is a breakdown of the diets that rounded out the top five in U.S. News and World Report's 2018 Best Diets ranking.

1:Mediterranean and DASH diets.

2:Flexitarian diet.

3:Weight Watchers.

4:MIND, TLC and Volumetrics diets.

5: MIND, TLC and Volumetrics diets.

3:What foods can you eat on the Mediterranean diet?

The Mediterranean diet emphasizes:

1:Eating primarily plant-based foods, such as fruits and vegetables, whole grains, legumes and nuts.

2:Replacing butter with healthy fats such as olive oil and canola oil.

3:Using herbs and spices instead of salt to flavor foods.

4:Limiting red meat to no more than a few times a month.

5:Eating fish and poultry at least twice a week.

6:Enjoying meals with family and friends .

7:Drinking red wine in moderation (optional) .

8: Getting plenty of exercise.

4:What should I eat if I want to lose weight?

1.Eat a high-protein breakfast.

2.Avoid sugary drinks and fruit juice.

3.Drink water a half hour before meals.

4.Choose weight loss-friendly foods.

5.Eat soluble fiber.

6.Drink coffee or tea.

7.Eat mostly whole, unprocessed foods.

8.Eat your food slowly.

9.Weigh yourself every day.

10.Get a good night's sleep, every night.

5:How can I reduce my stomach fat?

1:Eat Plenty of Soluble Fiber.

2:Avoid Foods That Contain Trans Fats.

3:Don't Drink Too Much Alcohol.

4:Eat a High-Protein Diet.

5:Reduce Your Stress Levels.

6:Don't Eat a Lot of Sugary Foods.

7:Do Aerobic Exercise (Cardio) .

8:Cut Back on Carbs, Especially Refined Carbs.

9: Replace Some of Your Cooking Fats With Coconut Oil.

10: Perform Resistance Training (Lift Weights).

11: Avoid Sugar-Sweetened Beverages.

12:Get Plenty of Restful Sleep.

13:Track Your Food Intake and Exercise.

14: Eat Fatty Fish Every Week.

15:Stop Drinking Fruit Juice.

16:Add Apple Cider Vinegar to Your Diet.

17:Eat Probiotic Foods or Take a Probiotic Supplement.

18: Try Intermittent Fasting.

19: Drink Green Tea.

20:Change Your Lifestyle and Combine Different Methods.

6:What is the most successful diet program?

The Top Diets to Try in 2018, According to Experts

1:DASH Diet.

2:Mediterranean Diet.

3:Flexitarian Diet.

4:Weight Watchers.

5:MIND Diet.

6:TLC Diet.

7:Volumetrics.

7:What foods can I eat on the whole30 diet?

What You Can Eat on Whole30

1:Vegetables. Eat vegetables — including potatoes! .

2:Fruits. Fruits are allowed, in moderation.

3:Unprocessed Meats. Sausage is still okay, but check for added sugar and other off-limit preservatives.

4:Seafood.

5:Eggs.

6:Nuts and seeds.

7:Oils (some) and ghee.

8:Coffee.

8:What's the most popular diet?

7 Popular Diets :

•The Ketogenic Diet.

•The Mediterranean Diet.

•The Paleo Diet.

•The Whole30 Diet.

•Weight Watchers Freestyle.

•The Vegan Diet.

•The Raw Food Diet.

9:What should you not eat when dieting?

1. French Fries and Potato Chips.

2. Sugary Drinks.

3. White Bread.

4. Candy Bars.

5. Most Fruit Juices.

6. Pastries, Cookies and Cakes.

7. Some Types of Alcohol (Especially Beer).

8. Ice Cream.

9.Pizza.

10. High-Calorie Coffee Drinks.

11. Foods High in Added Sugar.

10: How can I lose my stomach fat?

20 Effective Tips to Lose Belly Fat (Backed by Science):

1.Eat Plenty of Soluble Fiber.

2.Avoid Foods That Contain Trans Fats.

3.Don't Drink Too Much Alcohol.

4.Eat a High-Protein Diet.

5.Reduce Your Stress Levels.

6.Don't Eat a Lot of Sugary Foods.

7.Do Aerobic Exercise (Cardio) .

8.Cut Back on Carbs, Especially Refined Carbs.

9.Replace Some of Your Cooking Fats With Coconut Oil.

10.Perform Resistance Training (Lift Weights).

11.Avoid Sugar-Sweetened Beverages.

12.Get Plenty of Restful Sleep.

13. Track Your Food Intake and Exercise.

14. Eat Fatty Fish Every Week.

15. Stop Drinking Fruit Juice.

16. Add Apple Cider Vinegar to Your Diet.

17. Eat Probiotic Foods or Take a Probiotic Supplement.

18. Try Intermittent Fasting.

19. Drink Green Tea.

20.Change Your Lifestyle and Combine Different Methods.

11: What can I drink to burn belly fat?

15 foods and drinks that will help BLAST belly fat!

•Water.

•Apple cider vinegar.

•Chia seeds.

•Açai berries.

•Cinnamon.

•BCAAs.

•Green coffee.

•Green tea.

•Parsley.

•Celery.

•Spirulina.

•Healthy Mummy Smoothies.

•Wheatgrass.

•Yoghurt.

•Dandelion tea.

12: How can I lose my belly fat in 2 days?

Best Ways To Lose Belly Fat In 2 Days:

1.Consume 4 Meals A Day .

2.Eat Fat.

3.Sleep.

4.Take A 5-Minute After-Meal Walk.

5.Vitamin C.

6.Eat Slowly.

7.Sugar Is Your Opponent.

8.Limiting Carbohydrate Intake .

9. Say No To Gas Producing Vegetables.

13: What exercise burns the most belly fat?

Read on and burn the unwanted calories with these exercises to burn stomach fat quickly.

1: Running or walking.

2: Elliptical trainer.

3: Bicycling.

4: The bicycle exercise.

5: The Captain's chair leg raise.

6: Exercise ball crunch.

7: Vertical leg crunch. .

8: Reverse crunch.

14: How can I get a flat stomach in 3 days?

12 Ways To Make Your Belly Flatter By The End Of The Day:

1.Drink hot water and lemon.

2.Try a day going gluten-free or dairy-free.

3.Replace your usual snack with pineapple.

4.Keep an eye on your sodium intake.

5.Eat slower.

6.Stop chewing gum.

7.Stay away from fizzy drinks.

8.Eat more fibre.

9. Keep an eye on your portion sizes.

10.Avoid alcohol.

11.Drink peppermint tea.

12.Skip dessert .

15: How do you get a flat stomach in minutes?

Knee-Up with Overhead Press

1: Sit on mat with knees bent and feet on floor, holding dumbbells near shoulders, elbows by sides, palms in.

2: Lean back slightly and extend arms overhead as you lift feet a few inches off floor and bring knees toward chest.

3: Hold position for 1 to 3 counts; return to start. Do 15 reps.

16: How can I tone my stomach overnight?

12 Ways To Make Your Belly Flatter By The End Of The Day

1.Drink hot water and lemon.

2.Try a day going gluten-free or dairy-free.

3.Replace your usual snack with pineapple.

4.Keep an eye on your sodium intake.

5.Eat slower.

6.Stop chewing gum.

7.Stay away from fizzy drinks.

8.Eat more fibre.

9.Keep an eye on your portion sizes.

10.Avoid alcohol.

11.Drink peppermint tea.

12.Skip dessert.

17: How can I get my stomach flat fast?

Here are 30 science-backed methods to help you reach your goal of a flat stomach.

1.Cut Calories, but Not Too Much.

2.Eat More Fiber, Especially Soluble Fiber.

3.Take Probiotics.

4.Do Some Cardio.

5.Drink Protein Shakes.

6.Eat Foods Rich in Monounsaturated Fatty Acids.

7.Limit Your Intake of Carbs, Especially Refined Carbs.

8.Do Resistance Training.

9.Do Exercises Standing Instead of Sitting.

10.Add Apple Cider Vinegar to Your Diet.

11.Walk at Least 30 Minutes Each Day.

12.Avoid Liquid Calories.

13.Eat Whole, Single-Ingredient Foods.

14.Drink Water.

15. Practice Mindful Eating.

16.Avoid Swallowing Air and Gases.

17.Do High-Intensity Training.

18.Reduce Your Stress Levels.

19.Eat More Protein.

20.Track Your Food Intake.

21.Eat Eggs.

22.Get Enough Sleep.

23.Try Intermittent Fasting.

24.Eat Fatty Fish Every Week or Take Fish Oil.

25.Limit Your Intake of Added Sugar.

26.Replace Some Fat With Coconut Oil.

27.Strengthen Your Core.

28.Drink (Unsweetened) Coffee or Green Tea.

29. Don't Drink Too Much Alcohol.

30. Sneak Extra Activity Into Your Day.

18: How can I get a flat stomach in 30 days?

30-Day Countdown to a Flat Belly By Summer:

1.Do Some Flat Planks.

2.Sleep 7 to 8 Hours.

3.Snack On Popcorn.

4.Try Flutter Kicks And Criss Crosses.

5.Drink Water Before Each Meal.

6.Toss Some Berries And Nuts Into Your Oats.

7.Pair Split Lunges With Bicep Curls.

8.Cut Your Sugar Intake And IncreaseThe Amount Of Fiber You Eat.

9.Make Hummus Your Go-To Dip.

10.Experiment With Varied Cardio.

11.Stay Away From Stress.

12.Eat Eggs Instead Of Cereal.

13.Work A Medicine Ball Into Your Gym Routine.

14.Be Mindful.

15.Choose Greek Yogurt Over Regular Yogurt.

16.Build More Muscle Via Strength Training.

17.Know Your Go-To Foods.

18.Embrace Meatless Monday.

19.Try High-Intensity Interval Training.

20.Ditch Artificial Sweeteners.

21.Add Apple Cider Vinegar To Salad Dressings.

22.Hop On A Trampoline.

23.Ditch The Refined Grains.

24.Add Some Almonds To Your Salad.

25.Do Squats With A Bicycle Crunch.

26.Let Your Healthy Belly Bacteria Thrive.

27.Add Beans To Your Meals.

28.Just Dance!.

29.Snack Smart.

30.Use Avocado Instead Of Mayo On A Sandwich.

Chapter two

19: How can I get a flat tummy naturally?

11 Simple Ways to Reduce Belly Fat in 1 Week:

1: Eating Smaller Portions More Often.

2: Reduce Intake Of High-Fibre Foods.

3:Regulate Intake Of Raw Fruits And Veggies.

4:Cut Back On Dairy.

5:Eat More Potassium-Rich Foods.

6: Eat More Berries And Nuts.

7: Drink More Water.

8: Green Tea Helps.

9: Start Your Day With A Smoothie.

10: Make Ginger Your Friend.

11: Stay Away From Alcohol And Carbonated Drinks.

20: How can I tone my stomach fast?

5 Steps to Toning your Stomach:

1.: Cardio training and Strength Training.

2.: Abdominal exercises.

3.: Healthy eating.

4.: Avoid excess sodium, alcohol, and soda.

5.: Proper hydration.

21: What are the 5 foods that burn belly fat?

5 Foods That Banish Belly Fat

1: Oatmeal.

2: Blueberries. Research has shown that a diet rich in blueberries may help diminish belly fat.

3 : Almonds.

4 : Salmon.

5 : Lettuce.

22: How can I lose my gut in 2 weeks?

Here are 6 evidence-based ways to lose belly fat.

1.Don't eat sugar and avoid sugar-sweetened drinks.

2.Eating more protein is a great long-term strategy to reduce belly fat.

3.Cut carbs from your diet.

4.Eat foods rich in fiber, especially viscous fiber.

5.Exercise is very effective at reducing belly fat.

6.Track your foods and figure out exactly what and how much you are eating.

23: How can I get rid of my gut in 10 days?

1.Drink lots of water.

2.Cut down on carbs.

3.Increase protein intake.

4.Stay away from fad diets.

5.Eat slowly.

6.Walk, and then walk some more.

7.Crunches can save your day.

8.Take up a de-stressing activity.

9.Stay away from temptation.

10.Basic crunches.

11.Get more out of crunches.

24: How can I lose weight in 10 days?

How to Become Slim in 3 to 10 Days:

1.Drink Water. Start your day with a glass or two of plain water.

2.Walk After Your Meals. If you are not cut out for running or exercising then we might have something simpler for you.

3.Eat More Fiber. High-fiber foods are good for your health and weight loss.

4.Eat at Home.

5.Eat less Salt.

6.Run.

7.Do Push-ups/Squats

25: What are the 10 best exercises to lose weight?

Here 10 Best Exercises for Weight Loss:

•Lunges. There are many variations to the lunge, but the plain jane forward lunge is still very effective for weight loss, as it works multiple muscles at once (think: glutes, quads, and hamstrings) for max calorie burn.

•Burpees.

•Explosive Lunges.

•Squats.

•Double Jump.

•Mountain Climbers.

•Tabata Drill.

•Jump Rope.

26: What should I eat for breakfast to lose weight fast?

Eat These Foods for Breakfast to Lose Weight Faster:

•Avocado. Avocados go with everything, basically.

•Steel-cut oatmeal. So much better than Lucky Charms.

•Eggs and toast. An egg breakfast sandwich is both filling and delicious.

•Nut butter. Most nut butters are healthier than peanut butter.

•Spinach. There's a lot of protein packed into these leaves.

•Greek yogurt.

•Brown rice.

27: How can I reduce my tummy with exercise?

1: Crunches, Nothing burns belly fat faster than crunches, which occupy the number one position in fat-burning exercises.

2: Twist Crunches: Image: shutterstock.

3: Side Crunch: Image: shutterstock.

4: Reverse Crunches: Now it's time to do reverse crunches.

5: Vertical Leg Crunch .

6: Bicycle Exercise.

7: Lunge Twist.

8 : Rolling Plank Exercise

9: The Stomach Vacuum

10: Captain's Chair

11: Side To Side

28: What exercise burns the most calories in 30 minutes?

1.Running.

2.Strength Training.

3.Body Weight Workouts.

4.Interval Training.

5.Swimming.

29: Is it okay to exercise at night?

Specialists tend to disagree if exercise at night can be helpful or harmful to your health. Avoid sleeping right after working out because your metabolism will be accelerated, making it difficult to relax. Give yourself at least two hours to wind down before sleep and replenish your body with healthy foods.

30: How can I get rid of my gut in 2 weeks?

22 Ways to Lose 2 Inches of Belly Fat in 2 Weeks:

1.Start Your Day Early.

2.Eat More Antioxidants.

3.Avoid Hydrogenated Oils.

4.Switch to Sprouted Bread.

5.Lift Weights.

6.Stop Adding Sweeteners to Your Food and Drinks.

7.Eat More Fiber.

8.Swap Ketchup for Salsa.

9.Get More Vitamin D.

10.Eat More Nuts.

11.Try a High-Intensity Exercise Routine.

12.Flavor Your Food With Garlic.

13.Brush Your Teeth.

14.Eat More Omega-3s with Fish.

15.Keep Whole Grains in Your Diet.

16.Add Some Acid.

17.Snack on Veggies.

18.Crank Up the Calcium.

19.Snack on Tart Cherries.

20.Ramp Up Your Cardio Exercise.

21.Get More Sleep.

22.Avoid Eating After Dinner.

31: What foods burn fat the most?

12 Healthy Foods That Help You Burn Fat:

1.Fatty Fish. Fatty fish is delicious and incredibly good for you.

2.MCT Oil. MCT oil is made by extracting MCTs from coconut or palm oil.

3.Coffee. Coffee is one of the most popular beverages worldwide.

4.Eggs. Eggs are a nutritional powerhouse.

5.Coconut Oil.

6.Green Tea.

7.Whey Protein.

8.Apple Cider Vinegar

9.Chili Peppers

10.Oolong Tea

11.Full-Fat Greek Yogurt

12.Olive Oil

32: What veggies get rid of belly fat?

Here Are Some Of The Best Vegetables That You Can Include In Your Diet To Lose Belly Fat Quickly:

•Spinach And Other Leafy Greens.

•Mushrooms.

•Cauliflower And Broccoli.

•Chillies.

•Pumpkin.

•Carrots.

•Beans.

•Asparagus.

•Cucumbers

33: How can I burn fat naturally?

30 Easy Ways to Lose Weight Naturally (Backed by Science)

1.Add Protein to Your Diet. When it comes to weight loss, protein is the king of nutrients.

2.Eat Whole, Single-Ingredient Foods.

3.Avoid Processed Foods.

4.Stock Up on Healthy Foods and Snacks.

5.Limit Your Intake of Added Sugar.

6.Drink Water.

7.Drink (Unsweetened) Coffee.

8.Supplement With Glucomannan.

9.Avoid Liquid Calories

10. Limit Your Intake of Refined Carbs

11. Fast Intermittently

12.Drink (Unsweetened) Green Tea

13. Eat More Fruits and Vegetables

14. Count Calories Once in a While

15. Use Smaller Plates

16.Try a Low-Carb Diet

17.Eat More Slowly

18.Replace Some Fat with Coconut Oil

19.Add Eggs to Your Diet

20.Spice Up Your Meals

21.Take Probiotics

22.Get Enough Sleep

23.Eat More Fiber

24.Brush Your Teeth After Meals

25.Combat Your Food Addiction

26.Do Some Sort of Cardio

27.Add Resistance Exercises

28.Use Whey Protein

29.Practice Mindful Eating

30.Focus on Changing Your Lifestyle

34: What exercise gets rid of stomach fat?

Answer: Exercise alone will not do the job. Strengthening abdominal muscles can help you look tighter and thinner. But spot exercises won't banish belly fat. The real secret to losing belly fat is a balanced, calorie-controlled diet and an hour a day of moderate activity such as brisk walking.

35: How can I reduce my tummy in 30 days?

1.One, it's impossible to "spot reduce."

2.Follow an intermittent fasting eating routine.

3.Do some cardio first thing in the morning.

4.Do HIIT training at least three times a week.

5.Do some basic strength training.

6.Do a reasonable amount of core exercises.

7.Lose some weight.

36: How can I lose my belly fat in a week?

How to Lose Your Belly Fat Quickly and Naturally:

1.Stop Doing Crunches. Crunches will strengthen your stomach muscles, but won't burn the belly fat that covers your abs.

2.Get Stronger. Strength training builds muscle mass, prevents muscle loss and helps fat loss.

3.Eat Healthy.

4.Limit Alcohol Consumption.

5.Eat Less Carbs.

6.Eat More.

7.Eat More Protein.

8.Eat More Fat.

37: How much weight can I lose in a month?

At one to two pounds per week, losing 25 pounds will take you a little more than 12 weeks, or three months. To lose weight in a healthy manner, you should cut 500 to 1,000 calories a day by eating less and exercising more.

38: How can I lose fat quickly?

The 14 Best Ways to Burn Fat Fast

1.Start Strength Training. Strength training is a type of exercise that requires you to contract your muscles against resistance.

2.Follow a High-Protein Diet.

3.Squeeze in More Sleep.

4.Add Vinegar to Your Diet.

5.Eat More Healthy Fats.

6.Drink Healthier Beverages.

7.Fill up on Fiber.

8.Cut Down on Refined Carbs.

9.Increase Your Cardio

10.Drink Coffee

11.Try High-Intensity Interval Training (HIIT)

12. Add Probiotics to Your Diet

13.Increase Your Iron Intake

14.Give Intermittent Fasting a Shot

39: What foods help burn belly fat?

Eight Delicious Foods That Help Fight Belly Fat

•Avocados. Merely half of one avocado contains 10 grams of healthy mono-saturated fats, which stop the blood sugar spikes that tell your body to store fat around your midsection.

•Bananas.

•Yogurt.

•Berries.

•Chocolate Skim Milk.

•Green Tea.

•Citrus.

•Whole Grains.

40: Can hot water burn belly fat?

Therefore, a healthy diet alone is not enough. If you do not drink enough water, the food's nutrients will not go to other body parts. Other than this, water helps in the digestion of food and consequently, help burn more calories. This will lead to losing belly fat.

41:What can you do before bed to lose weight?

To lose weight, practice these 6 habits before bed

1.Eat a well-balanced meal for dinner. If you have a well-balanced meal full of carbs, protein, and fat, you'll feel full longer and won't go to bed hungry, Christman told Fox News.

2.Have a hot cup of herbal tea.

3.Stay busy.

4.Turn off your smartphone.

5.Find ways to relax.

6.Floss and brush your teeth.

42: Does apple cider vinegar burn belly fat?

According to this study, adding 1 or 2 tablespoons of apple cider vinegar to your diet can help you lose weight. It can also reduce your body fat percentage, make you lose belly fat and decrease your blood triglycerides.

43: How much weight can you lose in 2 days?

You will likely lose weight on any diet if you eat less than 910 calories a day. But losing 10 pounds in 3 days is both unlikely and unhealthy. To lose just 1 pound of body fat, you need to reduce your daily calories by about 500 a day for a whole week.

44: Can you lose belly fat?

Diet: There is no magic diet for belly fat. But when you lose weight on any diet, belly fat usually goes first. Getting enough fiber can help. Hairston's research shows that people who eat 10 grams of soluble fiber per day -- without any other diet changes -- build up less visceral fat over time than others.

45: How do you cure a bloated stomach?

Treatments to prevent or relieve bloating

1.Avoid chewing gum.

2.Limit your intake of carbonated drinks.

3.Avoid foods that cause gas, such vegetables in the cabbage family, dried beans, and lentils.

4.Eat slowly and avoid drinking through a straw.

5.Use lactose-free dairy products (if you are lactose intolerant)

Chapter three

46: How can I lose weight fast without exercise in a week?

11 Proven Ways to Lose Weight Without Diet or Exercise:

1.Chew Thoroughly and Slow Down. Your brain needs time to process that you've had enough to eat.

2.Use Smaller Plates for Unhealthy Foods.

3.Eat Plenty of Protein.

4.Store Unhealthy Foods out of Sight.

5.Eat Fiber-Rich Foods.

6.Drink Water Regularly.

7.Serve Yourself Smaller Portions.

8.Eat Without Electronic Distractions.

9.Sleep Well and Avoid Stress

10.Eliminate Sugary Drinks

11.Serve Unhealthy Food on Red Plates

47: Do Crunches burn fat?

This fat can come from anywhere in the body, and not just from the body part being exercised. Additionally, doing sit-ups and crunches isn't particularly effective for burning calories.

48: How much do I need to exercise to lose weight?

If you want to lose weight, shoot for at least 200 minutes (more than three hours) a week of moderate intensity exercise with everything else consistent, says Church. If you cut calories and exercise, he says, you can get away with a minimum dose of 150 minutes (2 1/2 hours) a week.

49: What causes abdominal fat?

Stress and Cortisol. Cortisol is a hormone that's essential for survival. It's produced by the adrenal glands and is known as a "stress hormone" because it helps your body to mount a stress response. Unfortunately, it can lead to weight gain when produced in excess, especially in the abdominal region.

50: How do you do crunches?

To isolate your abdominal muscles, lie on your back with your knees slightly bent. Make sure your feet are planted firmly on the floor and about hip-width-distance apart. Keep your knees comfortably apart. Fold your arms on your chest and tighten your abdominal muscles.

51: Can you shrink your stomach without surgery?

Once you are an adult, your stomach pretty much remains the same size -- unless you have surgery to intentionally make it smaller. Eating less won't shrink your stomach, says Moyad, but it can help to reset your "appetite thermostat" so you won't feel as hungry, and it may be easier to stick with your eating plan.

52: Why is my belly so bloated?

Bloating is when your belly feels swollen after eating (1). It is usually caused by excess gas production or disturbances in the movement of the muscles of the digestive system (2). Bloating can often cause pain, discomfort and a "stuffed" feeling. It can also make your stomach look bigger (3).

53: How much water should I drink to lose weight?

"It depends on your size and weight, and also on your activity level and where you live," Nessler says. "In general, you should try to drink between half an ounce and an ounce of water for each pound you weigh, every day." For example, if you weigh 150 pounds, that would be 75 to 150 ounces of water a day.

54: What does fish oil do?

Omega-3 fish oil contains both docosahexaenoic acid (DHA) and eicosapentaenoic acid (EPA). Omega-3 fatty acids are essential nutrients that are important in preventing and managing heart disease. Findings show omega-3 fatty acids may help to: Lower blood pressure.

55: What should I eat to get abs?

The Best Foods to Eat For Getting That Six-Pack:

1.Lean Protein. Josh suggests incorporating more lean, high-quality protein into your diet — think chicken breasts, fish and lean cuts of beef.

2.Nuts. As counter-intuitive as this sounds, fats are key for weight loss.

3.Yogurt.

4.Berries.

5.Quinoa.

6.Green Tea.

56: What is the fastest way for a kid to lose weight?

7 ways to help your child lose weight

1.Set realistic goals for your child. Because children are still growing, it may be a better to help them maintain rather than lose weight.

2.Encourage exercise.

3.Choose healthy and nutritious foods.

4.Change your family's eating habits.

5.Try behavior modification techniques.

6.Follow-up with your pediatrician.

7.Be supportive.

57: How do men get toned abs?

Flat Abs Exercise: Reverse Crunch. You can do the crunch in reverse by keeping your upper body flat on the ground while lifting your legs and lower torso, instead of the other way around. Here's how: Lay flat on your back with your knees bent and feet on the floor.

58: How many calories do I need a day?

An average woman needs to eat about 2000 calories per day to maintain, and 1500 calories to lose one pound of weight per week. An average man needs 2500 calories to maintain, and 2000 to lose one pound of weight per week. However, this depends on numerous factors.

59: How many calories are in a pound?

Because 3,500 calories equals about 1 pound (0.45 kilogram) of fat, it's estimated that you need to burn about 3,500 calories to lose 1 pound. So, in general, if you cut about 500 to 1,000 calories a day from your typical diet, you'd lose about 1 to 2 pounds a week.

60: Should you drink a gallon of water a day?

To prevent dehydration, you need to drink adequate amounts of water. There are many different opinions on how much water you should be drinking every day. Health authorities commonly recommend eight 8-ounce glasses, which equals about 2 liters, or half a gallon.

61: Does drinking water help lose weight?

The short answer is yes. Drinking water helps boost your metabolism, cleanse your body of waste, and acts as an appetite suppressant. Also, drinking more water helps your body stop retaining water, leading you to drop those extra pounds of water weight.

62: Can I drink too much water?

Although uncommon, it's possible to drink too much water. When your kidneys can't excrete the excess water, the sodium content of your blood is diluted (hyponatremia) — which can be life-threatening. In general, though, drinking too much water is rare in healthy adults who eat an average American diet.

63: How can I reduce my appetite permanently?

18 Science-Based Ways to Reduce Hunger and Appetite

1.Eat Enough Protein. Adding more protein to your diet can increase feelings of fullness, make you eat less at your next meal and help you lose fat (1, 2).

2.Opt for Fiber-Rich Foods.

3.Pick Solids Over Liquids.

4.Drink Coffee.

5.Fill Up on Water.

6.Eat Mindfully.

7.Indulge in Dark Chocolate.

8.Eat Some Ginger.

9.Spice Up Your Meals

10.Eat on Smaller Plates

11.Use a Bigger Fork

12.Exercise

64: Does starving yourself burn fat?

When you dramatically reduce your calorie intake, you will lose weight. But it can also cause all kinds of health problems, including muscle loss. Further, when you start fasting, your body goes into conservation mode, burning calories more slowly.

65: How can I starve myself to lose weight fast?

1.10 Easy Ways to Lose Weight Without Starving Yourself. Shred unwanted kilos without surviving on salad alone.

2.Always Eat A Big Breakfast. No more Fruit Loops–you want some protein and fat.

3.Eat More!

4.Just Say No To Starches.

5.Lift Weights.

6.Think Before You Eat.

7.But Have Fun Once In A While—or Once a Week.

8.Go Low-Carb.

9.Never, Ever Drink Sweetened Soda

10.Don't Fear Fat

66: Will I lose weight if I stop eating for 3 days?

You will likely lose weight on any diet if you eat less than 910 calories a day. But losing 10 pounds in 3 days is both unlikely and unhealthy. To lose just 1 pound of body fat, you need to reduce your daily calories by about 500 a day for a whole week. That's giving up 3,500 calories over the course of 7 days.

67: Will you lose weight by not eating?

But instead of losing weight they are gaining the weight. It sounds logical that if you eat less often you will lose weight. Not eating regularly lowers the body's metabolic rate decreasing calorie consumption. Not eating kicks our body into 'starvation mode' pushing our body to conserve food and store it as fat.

68: Are tummy trimmers effective?

Why use complex gym equipment when you can lose your belly fat with a tummy trimmer. This easy to use exercise tool reduces your belly fat and also improves your posture. Not only the belly area, the tummy trimmer also strengthens your chest, arms, hips and thighs.

69: Are sit ups good for your back?

One reason is that sit-ups are hard on your back — they push your curved spine against the floor and work your hip flexors, the muscles that run from the thighs to the lumbar vertebrae in the lower back.

70: How do I tone my back?

1.Stand with feet hip-width apart, holding dumbbells at sides.

2.Bend knees slightly and hinge forward at the hips, keeping the back flat, arms straight, and hands under shoulders.

3.Bend elbows and lift weights toward chest, keeping your arms close to your body (they should skim your side).

71: What should you not eat to lose belly fat?

8 Foods to Limit or Avoid to Lose Belly Fat

•Dairy. Some people suffer from lactose intolerance without knowing it.

•Potato chips. One step that will most likely help you shed unwanted weight around your belly is cutting out unhealthy snacking, especially on salty potato chips.

•Sodas.

•Baked goods.

•Fried foods.

•Processed carbohydrates.

•Sweeteners and added sugar.

•Alcohol.

72: How can I flatten my bloated stomach?

10 Flat Belly Tips

1.Avoid Constipation.

2.Rule Out Wheat Allergies or Lactose Intolerance.

3.Don't Eat Too Fast.

4.Don't Overdo Carbonated Drinks.

5.Don't Overdo Chewing Gum.

6.Watch Out for Sugar-Free Foods.

7.Limit Sodium.

8.Go Slow with Beans and Gassy Vegetables.

9.Eat Smaller Meals More Often.

10.Try Anti-Bloating Foods and Drinks.

73: Is it harder to lose weight after 40?

If you're over 40, you may have noticed that it's easier to gain weight -- and harder to lose it -- than it used to be. Changes in your activity level, eating habits, and hormones, and how your body stores fat all can play roles. But a few simple steps may help you slim down.

74: How can I drop 10 lbs fast?

Here are the 7 steps you should follow in order to lose 10 pounds in a week.

1.Eat Fewer Carbs and More Lean Proteins.

2.Eat Whole Foods and Avoid Most Processed Junk Foods.

3.Reduce Your Calorie Intake by Following These Tips (See List)

4.Lift Weights and Try High-Intensity Interval Training.

5.Be Active Outside of the Gym.

6.Intermittent Fasting Is Another Simple Way to Reduce Weight Quickly

7.Use These Tips to Reduce Water Retention

75: Can I lose 3 pounds in 3 days?

You will likely lose weight on any diet if you eat less than 910 calories a day. But losing 10 pounds in 3 days is both unlikely and unhealthy. To lose just 1 pound of body fat, you need to reduce your daily calories by about 500 a day for a whole week. That's giving up 3,500 calories over the course of 7 days.

76: Can you drink water on the military diet?

You can drink water and black coffee or tea, but no soda, milk, juice, or alcohol. Stick to the menu as much as you can. You're allowed to switch out some foods if you have food allergies or other dietary needs.

77: Is walking good for weight loss?

Physical activity, such as walking, is important for weight control because it helps you burn calories. If you add 30 minutes of brisk walking to your daily routine, you could burn about 150 more calories a day. So keep walking, but make sure you also eat a healthy diet.

78: How many times a week should I exercise to lose weight?

If you want to lose weight, shoot for at least 200 minutes (more than three hours) a week of moderate intensity exercise with everything else consistent, says Church. If you cut calories and exercise, he says, you can get away with a minimum dose of 150 minutes (2 1/2 hours) a week.

79: Can you lose weight with yoga?

"Regular yoga practice can influence weight loss, but not in the "traditional" sense of how we link physical activity to weight loss. Many yoga practices burn fewer calories than traditional exercise (e.g., jogging, brisk walking); however, yoga can increase one's mindfulness and the way one relates to their body.

80: Is peanut butter good for weight loss?

Researchers found that a diet that includes foods with high levels of monounsaturated fats like peanut butter can help people lose weight and prevent heart disease. But the fat in this diet was the good kind: "heart-healthy" monounsaturated fats, found in foods such as olives, nuts, avocados and peanut butter.

81: How can a beginner start losing weight?

Here are 10 more tips to lose weight even faster:

1.Eat a high-protein breakfast.

2.Avoid sugary drinks and fruit juice.

3.Drink water a half hour before meals.

4.Choose weight loss-friendly foods

5.Eat soluble fiber.

6.Drink coffee or tea.

7.Eat mostly whole, unprocessed foods.

8.Eat your food slowly.

9.Weigh yourself every day

10.Get a good night's sleep, every night

82: Can I lose 50 pounds?

To lose 50 pounds or more, you will want to begin by calculating how many calories you should be eating each day. And if you eat less than you burn, your body will use your reserve fuels, often times body fat, and cause you to lose weight.

83: Is 1500 calories a day enough?

Eating just 1,500 calories per day while following a regular exercise program will likely lead to a healthy weight loss. However, 1,500 calories per day is too low for some regular exercisers, especially those trying to maintain or gain weight.

84: Can a woman lose weight on 1200 calories a day?

On a daily diet of 1,200 calories, most everyone will lose weight. This simple calculation will give you a daily calorie goal that can help you lose a healthy 1 to 2 pounds per week.

85: Is eating 1200 calories a day bad?

Why Eating 1200 Calories a Day is Extremely Unhealthy. But oh, how eating a 1200 calorie diet is so, so wrong. Divide that number by 3 and that's 400 calories per meal. And for the majority of people, this minimal amount of energy [aka calories] is more than 1200 for the majority of people.

86: Can you live on 1200 calories a day?

A low-calorie diet is one that restricts your intake to 1,200 to 1,600 calories per day for men, and 1,000 to 1,200 calories per day for women. Less extreme diets are easier to follow, they interrupt normal daily activities less, and are less risky if you're over 50 or have other health problems.

87: Will I lose weight on 900 calories a day?

The 900-Calorie Diet. Some dieters who are not obese or who are slightly overweight may try to lose weight by eating 800 or 900 calories a day. For these reasons, it's generally not a good idea to follow fad diets or trendy weight-loss programs that provide only 900 calories a day or less.

88: Will I lose weight if I only eat 1000 calories a day?

Although it's recommended that you create a calorie deficit of 500 to 1,000 calories a day to lose 1 to 2 pounds a week, this rate may be too aggressive for some people. You may lose weight quickly on a 1,000-calorie diet, but the lost weight is mostly water and lean mass -- not fat.

89: Does eating 1200 calories a day work?

In short, this diet works. Eat fewer calories than you burn and your body can resort to burning your fat stores. "It is not recommended that a person go under 1,200 calories a day, since it is very hard to get enough nutrients like calcium, protein, and magnesium on a calorie level less than 1,200."

90: Is 500 calories a day enough?

Consuming 500 calories a day is not a healthy diet. Normally, eating anything below 1200 calories per day will make your body assume there's a food shortage. It's recommended to consume around 1200 - 1500 calories per day in an effort to lose weight.

91: How much weight will I lose on 800 calories a day?

A low-calorie diet is one that restricts your intake to 1,200 to 1,600 calories per day for men, and 1,000 to 1,200 calories per day for women. Some people go on a very low-calorie diet for rapid weight loss, often consuming only 800 calories a day.

Chapter four

92: Does Undereating cause weight gain?

Undereating is not the cause of your weight stall. Myth 3: I can never consume fewer than 1,200 calories or my body will go into starvation mode and weight loss will stop. Your body goes into "starvation" mode the minute you cut calories to lose weight.

93: Is 1200 calories a day too little?

As a general rule, people need a minimum of 1,200 calories daily to stay healthy. People who have a strenuous fitness routine or perform many daily activities need more calories. If you have reduced your calorie intake below 1,200 calories a day, you could be hurting your body in addition to your weight-loss plans.

94: What is a 1500 calorie diet?

1500 Calorie Diet Plan. Mix and match the meals for breakfast, lunch, dinner, and snack for a total of 1,500 calories a day. The 4-Week All-Over Makeover Diet. Get to your healthiest weight without feeling hungry, deprived, or bored. It's doable on this easy 1,500-calorie mix-and-match meal plan.

95: What happens if you only eat 1000 calories a day?

Although it's recommended that you create a calorie deficit of 500 to 1,000 calories a day to lose 1 to 2 pounds a week, this rate may be too aggressive for some people. You may lose weight quickly on a 1,000-calorie diet, but the lost weight is mostly water and lean mass -- not fat.

96: How much fat should I eat per day on a 1500 calorie diet?

For a daily 1,500-calorie diet, your DRI would be: Total fat: 33 to 58 grams. Total protein: 46 to 56 grams. Total carbohydrates: 130 grams

97: Is a 1200 calorie diet healthy?

Why Eating 1200 Calories a Day is Extremely Unhealthy. But oh, how eating a 1200 calorie diet is so, so wrong. Divide that number by 3 and that's 400 calories per meal. And for the majority of people, this minimal amount of energy [aka calories] is more than 1200 for the majority of people.

98: Can you lose weight by eating less and not exercising?

To lose weight, you need to eat less — not exercise more,. More exercise is unlikely to lead to more weight loss. Losing weight is a complicated process, but basically it comes down to creating an energy deficit — that is, burning more calories than you eat

99: How much carbs should I eat per day on a 1200 calorie diet?

It provides around 1200 calories a day, with about 30 to 45 grams of carbohydrate per meal, and 15 to 30 grams per snack.

100: Why do I not lose weight on 1200 calories a day?

If a 1,200-calorie diet creates more than a 1,000-calorie-per-day deficit and you're exercising on top of that, your body may slow down its calorie-burning processes because it senses starvation. Muscle burns more calories than fat, so your metabolism drops and it's harder to lose weight.

101: Will I lose weight eating 1200 calories a day without exercise?

Eat fewer calories than you burn and your body can resort to burning your fat stores. You lose weight as a result. "It is not recommended that a person go under 1,200 calories a day, since it is very hard to get enough nutrients like calcium, protein, and magnesium on a calorie level less than 1,200."

102: How do I stop starvation mode?

How to Avoid Starvation Mode & Support a Healthy Metabolism

1.Don't Cut Calories Too Low, Make Sure You Eat Enough!

2.Avoid Bingeing or Overeating by Eating Regularly.

3.Rest Enough and Avoid Overtraining.

4.Aim For Progress, Not Perfection.

103: What happens if I burn all the calories I eat?

If want to lose weight, consuming fewer calories than you burn daily helps you reach your goal. Eat 500 to 1,000 fewer calories than you burn daily to lose 1 to 2 pounds per week, suggests the Centers for Disease Control and Prevention.

104: Is 800 calories a day safe?

A low-calorie diet is one that restricts your intake to 1,200 to 1,600 calories per day for men, and 1,000 to 1,200 calories per day for women. Some people go on a very low-calorie diet for rapid weight loss, often consuming only 800 calories a day.

105: Is 1500 calories a day safe?

So now, your body is burning 1500 calories a day instead of 2000. Your body is actually even a little conservative so if you keep the deficit up too long it lowers even a bit more, say to 1400 calories per day (just to be safe)

106: Is 1000 calories a day too little?

Fast Weight Loss Is Unsustainable. Although it's recommended that you create a calorie deficit of 500 to 1,000 calories a day to lose 1 to 2 pounds a week, this rate may be too aggressive for some people. You may lose weight quickly on a 1,000-calorie diet, but the lost weight is mostly water and lean mass -- not fat.

107: Is 1000 calories a day enough for a woman?

In fact, a diet below 1,000 calories a day (called a very low-calorie diet or VLCD) increases your risk for gallstones and heart problems and should be followed only by obese people under a doctor's supervision. While you can drop to 1,200 calories per day and survive, doing so is not a smart idea.

108: Should you eat the calories you burn?

If you eat 2080 calories, then decide to add (eat) back 600 calories that you burned during exercise, you are now eating 2680 calories which is greater than your TDEE (more calories than your body can use). If you do this, you are no longer in a calorie deficit and burning fat. You are simply eating too many calories!

109: What happens if you only eat 500 calories a day?

Consuming 500 calories a day is not a healthy diet. Normally, eating anything below 1200 calories per day will make your body assume there's a food shortage. The end result will cause your body to go into what is known as "Starvation Mode". During this mode, your metabolism will slow down and try to conserve energy.

110: How can I lose 1 pound per day?

Steps :

1.Know the numbers. In order to lose one pound, you will need to burn 3,500 more calories than you consume in a day.

2.Reduce your caloric intake.

3.Keep a weight loss journal.

4.Get one to two hours of aerobic exercise every day.

5.Join an online fitness community.

6.Drink plenty of water.

7.Don't eat anything after 7:00pm.

111: How long should a diet break last?

Length and Frequency. 10-14 days, two weeks recommended. Unfortunately, some hormones simply take longer to recover to normal levels than others, so there is no cutting a diet break short.

112: How much weight will I lose eating 800 calories a day?

A low-calorie diet is one that restricts your intake to 1,200 to 1,600 calories per day for men, and 1,000 to 1,200 calories per day for women. Some people go on a very low-calorie diet for rapid weight loss, often consuming only 800 calories a day.

113: Is eating 900 calories a day bad?

The 900-Calorie Diet. Some dieters who are not obese or who are slightly overweight may try to lose weight by eating 800 or 900 calories a day. For these reasons, it's generally not a good idea to follow fad diets or trendy weight-loss programs that provide only 900 calories a day or less.

114: What is a reasonable amount of weight to lose in a month?

What According to the Centers for Disease Control and Prevention (CDC), it's 1 to 2 pounds per week. That means, on average, that aiming for 4 to 8 pounds of weight loss per month is a healthy goal. is a reasonable amount of weight to lose in a month?

115: Can you lose weight eating one meal a day?

The one meal a day diet is a weight loss plan that requires a person to eat only one meal per day. In the one meal a day diet, most people choose to not eat or drink anything with calories during the day.

116: Does the 5'2 diet really work?

The 5:2 diet is actually very simple to explain. For five days per week, you eat normally and don't have to think about restricting calories. Then, on the other two days, you reduce your calorie intake to a quarter of your daily needs. You should eat the same amount of food as if you hadn't been fasting at all.

117: What can you eat on the 5 2 diet?

Here are a few examples of foods that may be suitable for fast days:

•A generous portion of vegetables.

•Natural yogurt with berries.

•Boiled or baked eggs.

•Grilled fish or lean meat.

•Cauliflower rice.

•Soups (for example miso, tomato, cauliflower or vegetable)

•Low-calorie cup soups.

•Black coffee.

118: How much weight can you lose eating 800 calories a day?

A low-calorie diet is one that restricts your intake to 1,200 to 1,600 calories per day for men, and 1,000 to 1,200 calories per day for women. Some people go on a very low-calorie diet for rapid weight loss, often consuming only 800 calories a day.

119: What is the best diet plan to lose weight?

Here are 10 more tips to lose weight even faster:

•Eat a high-protein breakfast.

•Avoid sugary drinks and fruit juice.

•Drink water a half hour before meals.

•Choose weight loss-friendly foods (see list).

•Eat soluble fiber.

•Drink coffee or tea.

•Eat mostly whole, unprocessed foods.

•Eat your food slowly.

120: How much do you have to workout to lose a stone?

Do the math: You need to burn 3,500 calories to lose a pound. So if you're burning 300 calories in one workout, it will take you nearly 12 workouts to lose one pound. If you cut your calorie intake by 300 calories in addition to burning 300, it will take you half as long to lose a pound.

121: How does grapefruit burn fat?

Grapefruit can be part of a healthy weight loss diet because it's nutritious, not because of any mysterious fat-burning properties. A half grapefruit or a glass of grapefruit juice before meals may help fill you up, so you'll eat fewer calories at meals and potentially lose weight.

122: Is a starvation diet dangerous?

Dangers of Fasting for Weight Loss. When you dramatically reduce your calorie intake, you will lose weight. But it can also cause all kinds of health problems, including muscle loss. Further, when you start fasting, your body goes into conservation mode, burning calories more slowly.

123: Is the 5 bite diet safe?

Doctors suggests the 5-bite diet plan adds up to about 800 calories a day, which is less than half of generally recommended amounts, even for people trying to lose weight. The 5 Bite Diet is supposed to work like a gastric bypass without the surgery.

124: Can cutting calories help lose weight?

That's why cutting calories through dieting is generally more effective for weight loss. But doing both cutting calories through diet and burning calories through exercise can help give you the weight-loss edge. Exercise is also important because it can help you maintain your weight loss.

125: Which is better diet or exercise?

For most people, it's possible to lower their calorie intake to a greater degree than it is to burn more calories through increased exercise. That's why cutting calories through dieting is generally more effective for weight loss. Exercise is also important because it can help you maintain your weight loss.

126: How can I safely lose weight?

Here are 10 more tips to lose weight even faster:

1.Eat a high-protein breakfast.

2.Avoid sugary drinks and fruit juice.

3.Drink water a half hour before meals.

4.Choose weight loss-friendly foods .

5.Eat soluble fiber.

6.Drink coffee or tea.

7.Eat mostly whole, unprocessed foods.

8.Eat your food slowly.

9.Weigh yourself every day

10.Get a good night's sleep, every night.

127: What's a good diet plan?

A healthy eating plan:

1.Emphasizes vegetables, fruits, whole grains, and fat-free or low-fat dairy products.

2.Includes lean meats, poultry, fish, beans, eggs, and nuts.

3.Limits saturated and trans fats, sodium, and added sugars.

4.Controls portion sizes.

128: How many carbs should I eat daily to lose weight?

The dietary guidelines recommend that carbs provide 45 to 65 percent of your daily calorie intake. So if you eat a 2000-calorie diet, you should aim for about 225 to 325 grams of carbs per day. But if you need to lose weight, you will get much faster results eating around 50 to 150 grams of carbs.

129: How many calories should I eat to lose 2 pounds a week?

Because 3,500 calories equals about 1 pound (0.45 kilogram) of fat, it's estimated that you need to burn about 3,500 calories to lose 1 pound. So, in general, if you cut about 500 to 1,000 calories a day from your typical diet, you'd lose about 1 to 2 pounds a week.

130: What should I eat daily?

The pyramid, updated in 2005, suggests that for a healthy diet each day you should eat:

•6 to 8 servings of grains.

•2 to 4 servings of fruits and 4 to 6 servings of vegetables.

•2 to 3 servings of milk, yogurt, and cheese.

•2 to 3 servings of meat, poultry, fish, dry beans, eggs, and nuts.

131: How many calories does the average banana have?

A medium banana has 105 calories and 27 grams of carbohydrate. Not much more than many other types of fruit: 1 medium pear (103 calories, 27 gm carb), 1 medium apple (95 calories, 25 gm carb), 1 cup pineapple (82 calories, 21 gm carb) and 1 cup blueberries (84 calories, 21 gm carb).

132: What happens if you eat too few calories and work out?

The most effective way to lose weight is to consume fewer calories than you expend, creating a calorie deficit. But if your calorie intake dips too low, says Lummus, your body could go into starvation mode. Eating too few calories can be the start of a vicious cycle that causes diet distress.

133: How many calories are too few?

As a general rule, people need a minimum of 1,200 calories daily to stay healthy. People who have a strenuous fitness routine or perform many daily activities need more calories. If you have reduced your calorie intake below 1,200 calories a day, you could be hurting your body in addition to your weight-loss plans.

134: What does starvation mode mean?

Starvation mode implies that your body reduces calories out in an attempt to restore energy balance and stop you from losing any more weight, even in the face of continued calorie restriction. It involves a reduction in the amount of calories your body burns, which can slow down weight loss.

135: Can you exercise on a low calorie diet?

The fixed calorie diet plans don't work. If you go for fast weight loss you will not be able to sustain it for a long period unless you go extreme in the calorie reduction and exercise a lot. For people who have to lose more than 20 pounds (10kgs), the goal should be a loss of no more than 2 pounds or 1 kg per week.

136: Can you lose weight on 100 carbs a day?

50-100 Grams per Day. This range is great if you want to lose weight effortlessly while allowing for a bit of carbs in the diet. It is also a great range to maintain your weight if you are sensitive to carbs.

137: Is banana a carb?

Bananas generally contain between 72–135 calories and 19-35 grams of carbs, depending on their size. An average-sized banana contains about 100 calories and 25 grams of carbs.

138: What is the healthy amount of fat per day?

A standard low-fat diet contains about 30% of calories from fat, or less. Here are a few examples of suggested daily fat ranges for a low-fat diet, based on different calorie goals: 1,500 calories: About 50 grams of fat per day. 2,000 calories: About 67 grams of fat per day.

139: Are apples low carb?

The worst offenders are bananas, at 20 net carbs per 100 grams, and grapes, with 16 net carbs per 100 grams. But most fruits, including oranges and apples, are fairly high in sugar and carbs.

140: How many proteins should I eat daily?

The DRI (Dietary Reference Intake) is 0.8 grams of protein per kilogram of body weight, or 0.36 grams per pound. This amounts to: 56 grams per day for the average sedentary man.

141: Is 1600 calories a day healthy?

A low-calorie diet is one that restricts your intake to 1,200 to 1,600 calories per day for men, and 1,000 to 1,200 calories per day for women. Some people go on a very low-calorie diet for rapid weight loss, often consuming only 800 calories a day.

142: Can you survive on 1200 calories a day?

A low-calorie diet is one that restricts your intake to 1,200 to 1,600 calories per day for men, and 1,000 to 1,200 calories per day for women. Very low-calorie diets can help a person achieve weight loss of up to 3 to 5 pounds per week.

Chapter five

143: What should I stop eating to lose weight?

Here are 11 foods to avoid when you're trying to lose weight.

•French Fries and Potato Chips. Whole potatoes are healthy and filling, but french fries and potato chips are not.

•Sugary Drinks.

•White Bread.

•Candy Bars.

•Most Fruit Juices.

•Pastries, Cookies and Cakes.

•Some Types of Alcohol (Especially Beer)

•Ice Cream.

•Pizza

•High-Calorie Coffee Drinks

•Foods High in Added Sugar

144: Can you lose weight by not eating and just drinking water?

You don't eat and only drink water. Some water diets tell you to drink water for a few days, but let you add in fruits and vegetables once you've begun to lose weight. If you're a healthy person, a few days of fasting probably won't hurt you, according to Upton, but it's a bad way to lose weight.

145: Why do I not feel hungry?

Loss of Appetite. Hunger is your body's signal that it needs fuel. Your brain and gut work together to give you that feeling. So if you don't feel like eating, a number of things could cause that dip in appetite, including certain medications, emotions, and health issues.

146: Are eggs Low carb?

For those following a low carb diet, this day is the perfect holiday to celebrate because eggs are low in carbs while high in protein. This is another delicious egg recipe for breakfast that is very low in carbs it has 2.3 net carbs per serving. In fact, this recipe is approved for all phases of the Atkins diet.

147: How do I follow a low carb diet?

Eat: Meat, fish, eggs, vegetables, fruit, nuts, seeds, high-fat dairy, fats, healthy oils and maybe even some tubers and non-gluten grains. Don't eat: Sugar, HFCS, wheat, seed oils, trans fats, "diet" and low-fat products and highly processed foods.

148: Why do I lose more weight when not exercising?

One of the main reasons burning tons of calories through exercise can still result in not losing a single pound is because of an important thing you don't hear about very often from weight loss experts or the media. It's called inflammation. Too much exercise can cause inflammation in your body.

149: Why is my weight loss so slow?

During the first few weeks of losing weight, a rapid drop is normal. So as you lose weight, your metabolism declines, causing you to burn fewer calories than you did at your heavier weight. Your slower metabolism will slow your weight loss, even if you eat the same number of calories that helped you lose weight.

150: What medical conditions can stop you from losing weight?

Medical Reasons for Weight Gain

•Chronic stress .

•Cushing's syndrome .

•Hypothyroidism .

•Polycystic ovary syndrome (PCOS).

•Syndrome X.

•Depression .

•Hormonal changes in women.

151: Is there a medical reason I can t lose weight?

If it's underactive, you may have a condition called hypothyroidism. It can lead to weight gain from a buildup of salt and water in your body. An overactive thyroid is called hyperthyroidism. Many people with it lose weight, but others pick up extra pounds because it can make you feel hungrier.

152: How can I lose weight at 46?

Other Weight Loss Tips That Work:

1.Eat plenty of protein. Protein keeps you full and satisfied, increases metabolic rate and reduces muscle loss during weight loss (55, 56, 57).

2.Include dairy in your diet.

3.Eat foods high in soluble fiber.

4.Drink green tea.

5.Practice mindful eating.

153: What is the least amount of calories I can eat?

As a general rule, people need a minimum of 1,200 calories daily to stay healthy. People who have a strenuous fitness routine or perform many daily activities need more calories. If you have reduced your calorie intake below 1,200 calories a day, you could be hurting your body in addition to your weight-loss plans.

154: How can I reduce my metabolism?

Here are 6 lifestyle mistakes that can slow down your metabolism:

1.Eating Too Few Calories. Eating too few calories can cause a major decrease in metabolism.

2.Skimping on Protein.

3.Leading a Sedentary Lifestyle.

4.Not Getting Enough High-Quality Sleep.

5.Drinking Sugary Beverages.

6.A Lack of Resistance Training.

155: How long does it take for a person to starve to death?

Generally, it appears as though humans can survive without any food for 30-40 days, as long as they are properly hydrated. Severe symptoms of starvation begin around 35-40 days, and as highlighted by the hunger strikers of the Maze Prison in Belfast in the 1980s, death can occur at around 45 to 61 days.

156: What are the symptoms of starvation mode?

According to Clark, some of the signs and symptoms to look for which suggest there is some form of metabolic dysfunction include:

•Gas.

•Bloating.

•Constipation and/or diarrhoea.

•Reflux or heart burn.

•Low energy or fatigue.

•Increased hunger and food cravings.

•Reduced libido.

157: What does starvation do to the body?

Starvation is defined as a severe deficiency in caloric energy intake needed to maintain human life. In humans, prolonged starvation can cause permanent organ damage and eventually, death. The basic cause of starvation is an imbalance between energy intake and energy expenditure.

158: Does your body burn fat in starvation mode?

Starvation mode is a state in which the body responds to prolonged periods of low energy intake. During short periods of energy abstinence, the human body burns primarily free fatty acids from body fat stores, along with small amounts of muscle tissue to provide required glucose for the brain.

159: What happens if you burn more calories than you consume?

You gain weight when you eat more calories than you burn or burn fewer calories than you eat. While it is true that some people seem to be able to lose weight more quickly and more easily than others, everyone loses weight when they burn up more calories than they eat.

160: What happens if you burn 3500 calories a day?

Because 3,500 calories equals about 1 pound (0.45 kilogram) of fat, it's estimated that you need to burn about 3,500 calories to lose 1 pound. So, in general, if you cut about 500 to 1,000 calories a day from your typical diet, you'd lose about 1 to 2 pounds a week.

161: Should I burn more calories than I consume?

A calorie deficit is required for weight loss. This means you need to burn more calories than you consume. For many years, it was believed that a decrease of 3,500 calories per week would result in 1 lb (.45 kg) of fat loss. ... You may feel as though you're not eating very many calories.

162: Do you need to burn as many calories as you eat?

And if you eat fewer calories and burn more calories through physical activity, you lose weight. So, in general, if you cut about 500 to 1,000 calories a day from your typical diet, you'd lose about 1 to 2 pounds a week.

163: Can diarrhea cause weightloss?

Nutrition: Chronic diarrhea can cause you to become dehydrated, as your body loses too much fluid. And, chronic diarrhea can also result in weight loss if you aren't absorbing enough carbohydrates and calories from the food you eat.

164: Is it bad to count calories?

Is counting calories a good thing or is it bad for my health? It's always good to be aware of the amount and quality of the food you're eating, especially with overweight and obesity becoming more and more of a problem. That doesn't mean you need to pick up everything you eat and count the calories, though.

165: How much weight do I need to notice?

For a weight change to show up on your face, you'd need to change your BMI by 1.33 points, the study found. That means a woman and man of average height would need to gain or lose eight pounds and nine pounds, respectively.

166: How do you know if you are eating too little?

Here are 9 signs that you're not eating enough.

1.Low Energy Levels. Calories are units of energy your body uses to function.

2.Hair Loss. Losing hair can be very distressing.

3.Constant Hunger.

4.Inability to Get Pregnant.

5.Sleep Issues.

6.Irritability.

7.Feeling Cold All the Time.

8.Constipation.

9.Anxiety

167 : Is 1400 calories too low?

Most women should be able to lose 1-2lbs a week by restricting their daily calorie intake to 1,400 calories, and most men should be able to lose weight on 1,800 calories. If you're following a 1,400- calorie diet you should aim for around 300 calories for breakfast, 350 for lunch and 500 for your evening meal.

168: Are weight loss plateaus real?

According to the experts, hitting these plateaus is nothing unusual. As your weight drops and your body composition changes, so do your nutritional needs. There are several reasons why your weight can hit a plateau: As your weight goes down, you not only lose fat but also a small amount of muscle.

169: What is a reasonable weight loss goal?

Setting Reasonable Goals for Losing Weight. To prevent metabolic rebound, set a realistic goal of losing weight at a rate of about one pound a week. Remember that one pound of fat is equal to about 3,500 calories, and you need to cut that amount from your diet or burn it off through exercise to lose one pound.

170: What foods fill you up but are low in calories?

Here are 13 low-calorie foods that are surprisingly filling:

•Oats. Share on Pinterest.

•Greek Yogurt. Greek yogurt is a great source of protein that can help curb cravings and promote weight loss.

•Soup.

•Berries.

•Eggs.

•Popcorn.

•Chia Seeds.

•Fish.

171: Does apple cider vinegar help lose weight?

adding 1 or 2 tablespoons of apple cider vinegar to your diet can help you lose weight. It can also reduce your body fat percentage, make you lose belly fat and decrease your blood triglycerides.

172: How can I get fit?

The experts offer some other tips for home exercisers:

1.Challenge yourself and avoid boredom.

2.Find an exercise partner.

3.Schedule your workouts.

4.Use a journal to track your progress and jot down any breakthroughs you may have.

5.Set goals, like training for a race or losing 20 pounds.

173: Is diet or exercise more important for heart health?

Diet and exercise are an important part of your heart health. If you don't eat a good diet and you don't exercise, you are at increased risk of developing health problems. These include high blood pressure, high cholesterol, obesity, type 2 diabetes, and heart disease.

174: How do cleans eat for beginners?

Eating Clean For Beginners: 8 Guidelines:

1.Cook your own food.

2.Read the nutrition labels.

3.Eat whole foods.

4.Avoid processed foods.

5.Eat well-balanced meals.

6.Limit added fat, salt, and sugars.

7.Eat 5-6 meals per day.

8.Don't drink your calories.

175: How do I mentally prepare myself to lose weight?

Ask yourself why you want to lose weight. Keep these reasons in the forefront of your mind throughout your diet. Think about how you're motivated, and set up rewards (non-food) that help you stay on track. Include weekly rewards that will motivate you, and ask a friend to be your diet buddy.

176: How do I stay committed to lose weight?

Consider following these six strategies for weight-loss success.

1. Make a commitment. Long-term weight loss takes time and effort — and a long-term commitment.

2.Find your inner motivation. No one else can make you lose weight.

3.Set realistic goals.

4.Enjoy healthier foods.

5.Get active, stay active.

6.Change your perspective.

177: How do I keep myself motivated to lose weight?

16 Ways to Motivate Yourself to Lose Weight

1.Determine Why You Want to Lose Weight. Clearly define all the reasons you want to lose weight and write them down.

2.Have Realistic Expectations.

3.Focus on Process Goals.

4.Pick a Plan That Fits Your Lifestyle.

5.Keep a Weight Loss Journal.

6.Celebrate Your Successes.

7.Find Social Support.

8. Make a Commitment.

9.Think and Talk Positively

10.Plan for Challenges and Setbacks

11.Don't Aim for Perfection and Forgive Yourself

12.Learn to Love and Appreciate Your Body

13.Find an Exercise You Enjoy

14.Find a Role Model

15.Get a Dog ,dogs can increase your physical activity

16.Get Professional Help When Needed

178: How do I prepare my body to lose weight?

Create a meal plan that fits your lifestyle.

1.Include at least four to six servings of vegetables and fruit.

2.Focus on eating nutrient-dense foods.

3.Limit high-sugar foods and saturated fats, and reduce sodium intake.

4.Cut or reduce alcohol consumption to two drinks a week.

5.Avoid eating late in the day.

179: How do you stay mentally strong when losing weight?

Get that overweight mentality out of your head and start thinking like a thin person with these eight strategies:

1.Picture Yourself Thin. If you want to be thin, picture yourself thin.

2.Have Realistic Expectations.

3.Set Small Goals.

4.Get Support.

5.Create a Detailed Action Plan.

6.Reward Yourself.

7.Ditch Old Habits.

8.Keep Track.

180 : What color stimulates appetite?

While blue is considered an appetite-suppressing color, researchers often point to warm colors as appetite-stimulating. According to the Rohm and Haas Paint Quality Institute, red is a powerful color that increases blood pressure and heart rate.

181: Why do people eat for psychological reasons?

Emotional eating is responding to feelings such as stress by eating high-carbohydrate, high-calorie foods with low nutritional value. When untreated, emotional overeating can cause obesity, problems with weight loss, and even lead to food addiction.

182: How do you get your mind to lose weight?

1.Change Your Goals. Losing weight might be a result, but it shouldn't be the goal.

2.Rethink Rewards and Punishments.

3.Take a Breath.

4.Throw Out the Calendar.

5.Identify Your 'Trouble Thoughts'

6.Don't Step on the Scale.

7.Talk to Yourself Like You Would a Friend.

8.Forget the Whole 'Foods Are Good or Bad' Mentality.

183 : Is overeating genetic?

Overeating could be genetic, scientists believe, after discovering that an obesity gene causes people to eat too much. Previous studies had linked the gene to being overweight but scientists were unsure as to its effect on the body. The new study shows that it affects feelings of fullness after eating.

184: What affects what we eat?

The key driver for eating is of course hunger but what we choose to eat is not determined solely by physiological or nutritional needs. Some of the other factors that influence food choice include: Biological determinants such as hunger, appetite, and taste. Economic determinants such as cost, income, availability.

185: What factors have been the greatest influences on your eating behaviors?

Healthy Eating: Influences on Eating Behaviour

•Food is everywhere. For most people, it is easy to find something to eat, especially unhealthy options.

•Routines. Plan to eat, and make family meals routine.

•Marketing.

•Cultural and social meanings.

•Family and living situations.

•Emotions.

•Knowledge of nutrition,and Timing.

186: Can dancing lose belly fat?

Dance Moves to Help You Lose Belly Fat. Have fun blasting belly fat by dancing your way slim. And because the combination of cardio and strength exercise when paired with a healthy diet is key to losing body fat, dancing can be your new go-to workout for both fun and fitness.

187: How much weight can you lose by dancing?

One hour of fast dancing burns 446 calories if you weigh 155 pounds and 532 calories if you weigh 185 pounds. You need to burn 3,500 calories to lose 1 pound, so with three one-hour Zumba sessions a week, you should lose at least 1 pound in a little over two weeks or almost 2 pounds a month.

188: Which dance is best for weight loss?

Here are some dance forms that could trigger weight loss, make you more flexible, and give you that perfectly toned and sculpted body.

•Zumba. Zumba involves dance and aerobic movements performed to energetic music thereby giving you a perfect cardio workout.

•Belly dance.

•Hip hop.

•Salsa.

•Indian classical dance forms.

189: Is dancing better than walking?

In most cases, you'll burn more calories performing aerobic dance than walking on a treadmill. Intensity matters, however, and a vigorous power walk will torch more calories than a moderate dance session.

190: Does walking in place burn belly fat?

While any exercise can burn calories, brisk walking for 45 minutes mobilizes the body to dip into fat reserves and burn stored fat. It is especially good for burning internal belly fat, called visceral fat, that not only contributes to your waistline but also raises your risks for diabetes and heart disease.

191: Does Compression clothing help lose weight?

Your compression garments may accelerate weight loss through increased sweating. Most compression or tight-fitting clothing can make you sweat in the area you wear them, it may just help with that water weight loss that is often the first line of weight loss.

192: Do Body Shapers work to lose weight?

Do Body Shapers Help You Lose Weight During Exercise? ... Since body shapers make it more difficult to breathe, it might seem like you would burn more calories during exercise due to the increased stress on your body. But in reality, wearing a body shaper during a workout can do more harm than good.

193: How much weight can you lose in a sauna?

Because the intense heat makes you sweat, you'll lose excess water stored in your body. You can lose up to five pounds in a single session but, as you rehydrate, most of the weight will come back. However, if you need to shed a couple of pounds quickly, a sauna can help.

194: How long should you stay in a steam room to lose weight?

Sitting in the room makes you sweat copiously. Water lost through sweating contributes to the weight loss. You have effectively lost water weight and not fat. Steam bath for a duration of 30-45 minutes is said to decrease up to 5 pounds.

195: Do saunas burn fat?

Can You Lose Weight in a Sauna or Steam Room? Yes. But you're not building muscle, you aren't burning a significantly raised rate of calories, and you're really only losing water weight. In addition, not replacing the water you are sweating out can actually make it harder for your body to lose weight.

196: How long should I sit in the sauna?

Your first session should probably be no longer than 10 minutes. Taking a sauna is not a competitive sport and there is nothing to be gained by trying to stay in longer than you feel is comfortable. After 10 minutes, get out, take a cool shower and then go back in for another session of perhaps the same amount of time.

197: Can relaxing help you lose weight?

Meditation/Relaxation for Weight Loss. You may be surprised to hear that in addition to practicing yoga asanas, yoga relaxation and Yoga Sound Meditation can also help you lose weight. Stress may also cause the body to hold onto fat, making it harder to lose weight.

198: How can I lose weight while I sleep?

Incredibly, research suggests certain habits and a good night's sleep could make it easier to lose weight.

1.Before You Climb Into Bed.

2.Sleep in a Dark Room.

3.Use Your Air Conditioner.

4.Don't Sleep With Your Phone or Television.

5.A Good Night's Sleep Means Burning More Calories.

199: Why is it so hard for me to lose weight?

At the heart of weight gain is the hormone, insulin. One of the main reasons why so many people struggle to lose weight is not because they are idle or greedy but because their muscles have become resistant to insulin. But if you are "insulin resistant" then your muscles find it hard to absorb these calories.

200: Is sex good for weight loss?

The truth is that having sex could improve your chances of losing weight. Having sex can also reduce your food cravings and help you lose weight. Having sex burns calories. Eating healthy foods and exercising will increase your sex drive.